Health Psychology for Teenage Girls
Nutrition, Exercise, and Well-being

By
Chris Jorden

Table of Contents

Chapter 01
The Foundations of Nutrition: Recognizing the Significance of Micronutrients and Macroscopic Nutrients

Chapter 02
Eating for Energy: The Effects of Food Selection on Mood and Energy Levels

chapter 03
The Teenage Diet: Common Nutritional Challenges and How to Overcome Them

chapter 04
Healthy Eating on a Budget: Practical Tips for Affordable and Nutritious Meals

Chapter 05
Emotional Eating: Understanding the Connection Between Emotions and Food

chapter 06
Body Image and Nutrition: How Body Image Influences Eating Habits

chapter 07
Eating Disorders: Recognizing the Signs and Seeking Help

Chapter 08
Balanced Eating for Busy Teens: Strategies for Eating Well with a Busy Schedule

Chapter 9
How to Meet Your Nutritional Needs Without Eating Meat or Using Animal Products

chapter 10
Nutrition for Athletic Performance: Fueling the Body for Sports and Physical Activity

chapter 11
Mindful Eating: Techniques for Eating with Awareness and Enjoyment

chapter 12
Food and Mood: How Diet Affects Mental Health and Well-being
First of all,
chapter 13
Nutritional Supplements: Understanding When and How to Use Supplements Safely
chapter 14
Eating for Healthy Skin: Foods that Promote Clear, Healthy Skin
chapter 15
Gut Health and Nutrition: The Gut-Brain Connection and Its Impact on Overall Health
Chapter 16
Cooking and Food Preparation Skills: Fundamental Cooking Techniques for Nutritious Dinners

chapter 17:
Smart Snacking: Nutritious Snack Options for Long-Term Energy

chapter 18
Hydration: The Importance of Water and Staying Hydrated
chapter 19:
Eating Out Healthily: Making Healthy Choices
chapter 20: Understanding the Physical and Mental Benefits of Exercise and Its Role in Health
Chapter 21:
Conscientious Time Management: Allocating Time for What Really Counts
chapter 22
Overcoming Exercise Barriers: Dealing with Typical Challenges to Maintaining an Active Lifestyle
chapter 23

4

Establishing a Lifestyle that Encourages Good Food and Exercise Habits and Creating a Supportive Environment

Chapter 01
The Foundations of Nutrition: Recognizing the Significance of Micronutrients and Macroscopic Nutrients

Understanding the fundamentals of nutrition is essential for young females as they transition through puberty, as it is the cornerstone of health. We will dig into the realm of macronutrients and micronutrients in this chapter, examining their functions, origins, and significance in upholding a nutritious diet and way of life. Macronutrients are those nutrients that give off calories, which is how energy is obtained. They consist of lipids, proteins, and carbs, each of which has a specific function in the body. The body uses carbohydrates as its main energy source, especially for the muscles and brain. Foods including bread, pasta, grains, fruits, and vegetables all contain them. Glucose, the source for energy, is produced when carbohydrates are broken down. It's critical that teenage girls eat enough carbohydrates to fuel their expanding bodies and active lifestyles.

Proteins: Body tissues require proteins for development, maintenance, and repair. Amino acids, the building blocks of protein, make up what they are. Adolescent females, particularly those going through puberty, must consume enough protein. Macronutrients are those nutrients that offer calories for energy. Carbohydrates, proteins, and lipids are among them; each has a distinct function in the body.

Carbohydrates: The body uses them mostly for energy, especially the muscles and brain. Bread, pasta, grains, fruits, and vegetables are among the foods that contain them. Glucose, which is utilized as an energy source, is produced when carbohydrates are broken down. In order to maintain their developing bodies and active lifestyles, teenage females must eat enough carbohydrates.

Proteins: Growth, maintenance, and repair of biological tissues depend on proteins. The building components of protein are amino acids, which make them up. Adolescent girls must consume enough protein, especially when going through puberty. Micronutrients: The Powerful Assists

Micronutrients are necessary nutrients that are needed in trace amounts but are vital to many physiological functions.

Vitamins: Vitamins are organic substances that the body needs for a number of different biochemical processes. Water-soluble vitamins (such vitamin C and the B vitamins) and fat-soluble vitamins (including vitamins A, D, E, and K) are the two groups into which they are divided. Every vitamin has a distinct purpose that supports different aspects of the body, such as the immune system, bone health, vision, and antioxidant defense.

Minerals are inorganic substances that are necessary for a number of bodily physiological functions. They consist of trace minerals including iron, zinc, copper, selenium, iodine, and chromium as well as microminerals like calcium, magnesium, phosphorus, sodium, potassium, and chloride. Minerals for a number of bodily physiological functions. They consist of trace minerals including iron, zinc, copper, selenium, iodine, and chromium as well as macro minerals like calcium, magnesium, phosphorus, sodium, potassium, and chloride. Minerals play a variety of roles in the body, including maintaining fluid balance, neuron function, muscle contraction, bone health, and oxygen delivery.

The Value of Variety and Balance

It takes a balanced, diverse diet that offers an adequate intake of macronutrients and micronutrients to achieve optimal health and well-being. Every vitamin has a distinct function in maintaining general health, and imbalances or deficiencies can have a negative impact on health. All food groups are represented in a balanced diet, which includes a range of foods such as fruits, vegetables, whole grains, lean meats, and healthy fats. Teenage girls may make sure they get all the necessary elements required for growth, development, and vitality by eating a varied variety of foods.

All nutrients are necessary for good health, but moderation is the key. The health effects of consuming too much or too little of a certain nutrient might be detrimental. Adolescent females ought to strive for balance. and harmony in their diet, giving natural, nutrient-dense meals priority over processed foods, sugar-filled drinks, and bad fats. Variety is essential for optimum nutrition as well as being the flavor of life. Teenage girls can make sure they get a diversified assortment of nutrients necessary for overall health and well-being by eating a wide selection of meals from different food categories. Their palate can be expanded and new sources of important nutrients can be provided by experimenting with different foods and recipes.

In summary

In conclusion, young females must grasp the fundamentals of nutrition in order to make wise decisions regarding their food and way of life. They can feed their bodies optimally for growth, development, and vitality by understanding the roles and significance of macronutrients and micronutrients. The cornerstone of good health is a varied and balanced diet that offers an appropriate intake of all necessary elements. , supporting physical, mental, and emotional well-being. promoting mental, emotional, and physical well.

Chapter 02
Eating for Energy: The Effects of Food Selection on Mood and Energy Levels

➢ Food is more than simply nutrition; it plays a major role in regulating our mood and energy levels throughout the day.
➢ Our bodies use a variety of nutrients in a complicated process to turn the food we eat into energy.
➢ Eating the correct foods can assist maintain energy levels and encourage happiness.
➢ On the other hand, poor dietary decisions might cause mood and energy swings.
➢ Our energy and mood are influenced by the kinds of food we eat, when we eat them, and how much of them.
➢ A diet high in full, nutrient-dense foods can help maintain a stable mood and offer long-lasting energy.
➢ A diet heavy in processed foods and added sweets, however, can cause energy slumps and fluctuations in mood.
➢ Stable energy levels depend on the proper balance of macronutrients such proteins, lipids, and carbs. The body uses carbohydrates as its main energy source, and because they affect serotonin levels, they can have an effect on mood.
➢ Proteins are necessary for neurotransmitter activity, which influences mood and energy levels, and muscle repair.
➢ Fats have an impact on brain function, can elevate mood, and increase vitality.
➢ Energy and attitude are also greatly impacted by hydration, since even moderate dehydration can cause irritation and weariness.

➢ In order to prevent energy dumps, eating frequent meals and snacks can assist maintain steady blood sugar levels.
➢ Limiting sugar and caffeine intake can help avoid energy surges and crashes that can have an impact on mood.
➢ Including more foods high in fiber in your diet can help control blood sugar levels, increase feelings of fullness, and provide you with long-lasting energy.
➢ certain vitamins and Minerals that are important for energy production and mood modulation include magnesium, iron, and B vitamins.
➢ You can be sure you're getting all the nutrients required for the best possible energy and mood by eating a balanced diet that consists of a variety of foods.
➢ Eating mindfully, or observing your body's signals of hunger and fullness, might help you avoid overindulging and have more energy.
➢ A healthy gut microbiota can have a good effect on mood and energy levels, which highlights the importance of the gut-brain relationship. Ultimately, you can feel your best all day long by making wise food choices and being aware of how different foods affect your energy and attitude.

Eating for energy involves making meal choices that promote general health and wellbeing and give sustained energy throughout the day, rather than merely absorbing calories. This chapter examines the relationship between dietary choices and mood as well as how to maintain appropriate energy levels through nutrition. Our diets provide us with energy, mostly in the form of proteins, lipids, and carbs. The body prefers to use carbohydrates because they can be quickly transformed into glucose, which powers our cells. In addition to being necessary for the absorption of fat-soluble vitamins and the maintenance of cell structure, fats offer a concentrated source of energy. Although proteins are essential for the construction and repair of tissues, they are not the main source of energy until prolonged fasting or vigorous exercise are involved.

How Carbohydrates Affect Energy Levels: Sugars and other simple carbs give you a rapid energy boost, but they can also cause energy dumps. Because they contain more fiber, complex carbohydrates—found in whole grains, fruits, and vegetables—offer a more gradual release of energy. Including a combination of Meals containing both basic and complex carbohydrates can support steady energy levels all day long.

Fast's Function in the Production of Energy: For long-lasting vitality and general health, one needs healthy fats, including those in avocados, nuts, seeds, and olive oil. Flaxseeds, walnuts, salmon, and other fatty fish are good sources of omega-3 fatty acids, which are especially good for the brain and mood.

Proteases for Long-Term Energy: In addition to being necessary for the synthesis of energy, proteins are also involved in the maintenance and repair of tissues. Lean protein foods like turkey, chicken, fish, and beans can help keep blood sugar levels steady and encourage fullness throughout meals.

The Effect of Micronutrients on Mood and Energy Levels: Micronutrients, including vitamins and minerals, are necessary for the body to produce energy and control mood. Whole grains, meat, fish, and leafy greens are good sources of B vitamins, which are essential for turning food into energy. For the transportation of oxygen and the synthesis of energy, minerals like iron, which can be found in red meat, chicken, lentils, and spinach, are crucial. **Energy and Hydration Levels:** Energy levels can drop and weariness can result from dehydration. It's crucial to stay hydrated throughout the day in order to sustain general health and energy levels at their best.

Timing of Meals and Energy Levels: Consuming meals and snacks on a regular basis will help keep blood sugar levels constant and stave off energy dumps. Meals that contain fiber, protein, and healthy fats might help delay digestion and give you energy for longer.

The Effects of Sugar and Caffeine on Energy Levels: Although sugar and caffeine might give you a quick energy boost, they can also cause mood swings and energy dips. The detrimental effects of these drugs on energy levels can be lessened by consuming them in moderation and in combination with other nutrients. Eating mindfully, which includes observing your body's signals of hunger and fullness, might help you avoid overindulging and have more energy. Eating may be made more enjoyable and mood-boosting by taking the time to appreciate and enjoy meals.

Useful Advice on Consuming Food for Energy: Select whole, high-nutrient foods over processed ones. Include a range of nutritious grains, fruits, vegetables, lean meats, and healthy fats in your meals and snacks. Consume regular meals and snacks to keep your blood sugar levels steady. Drink plenty of water throughout the day. For long-lasting energy, cut back on sugar and caffeine intake and combine them with other nutrients. To improve your dining experience and your energy levels, practice mindful eating.

In summary

Making wise dietary choices that promote long-lasting energy levels and general wellbeing is the essence of eating for energy. Teenage girls can maximize their mood and energy levels all day long by practicing mindful eating, drinking plenty of water, and including a range of nutrient-dense foods in their meals and snacks.

chapter 03
The Teenage Diet: Common Nutritional Challenges and How to Overcome Them

Adolescence is a critical time for growth and development, therefore eating a healthy diet is important for overall health and wellbeing. However, a lot of youngsters deal with typical nutritional issues that, if left untreated, may negatively affect their health. This chapter examines these issues and offers doable solutions to help you keep your adolescent diet nutritious. Due to hectic schedules, a lot of youngsters skip meals or eat infrequently, which can result in energy imbalances and vitamin shortages. Teens are frequently lured to processed, convenient foods that are poor in nutrients but rich in sugar, salt, and harmful fats. Eating a repetitive diet deficient in vital nutrients might be caused by having few food options. Consuming large amounts of fast food or sugar-filled beverages might result in poor eating patterns due to peer pressure. In an effort to attain a particular body ideal, some teenagers may participate in improper dieting or restrictive eating, which can result in nutrient shortages and disordered eating patterns.

Methods for Overcoming Nutritional Obstacles

i. Creating Consistent Eating Routines: Encouraging teenagers to eat at regular intervals will help keep blood sugar levels constant and curb overindulgence.

ii. Promoting Balanced Meals: By highlighting the significance of incorporating a range of foods from every dietary group into meals, teens can be certain to receive all the vital nutrients required for healthy growth and development.

iii. Encouraging teenagers to select nutritious snacks like fruits, vegetables, nuts, and yogurt can help curb overindulgence and supply vital nutrients.
iv. Nutrition Education: Teenagers can make better decisions if they are informed about the value of nutrition and how to choose wholesome foods.
v. Promoting Family Meals: Sharing meals as a family can help to foster good eating practices and present chances for teenagers.

Typical Adolescent Nutritional Deficiencies

Iron: Because of menstrual blood loss, teenage girls are susceptible to iron deficiency. Foods high in iron, like beans, chicken, fish, red meat, and fortified cereals, can help ward off iron deficiency.
Calcium: For the growth and development of their bones, teenagers require calcium. Fortified meals, leafy green vegetables, and dairy products are excellent sources of calcium.
Vitamin D: Maintaining healthy bones need vitamin D. Vitamin D deficiency can be avoided by going outside and eating foods high in the nutrient, such as fatty fish and fortified meals.
Omega-3 Fatty Acids: The development and health of the brain depend on omega-3 fatty acids. Walnuts, flaxseeds, and fatty fish are excellent providers of omega-3 fatty acids.

Helpful Hints for Adolescents to Enhance Their Nutrition: Ensuring that kids have access to wholesome food throughout the day can be achieved by arranging meals and snacks in advance. Equipping youngsters with this skill will enable them to make well-informed dietary decisions. Encouraging teenagers to cook at home can help them try different foods and form good eating habits. Maintaining your general health and energy levels during the day can be achieved by drinking lots of water. Be Aware of Portion Sizes: Educating youngsters on sensible serving sizes will help curb overindulgence and encourage a diet rich in nutritious foods.

In summary

For the purpose of forming lifelong healthy eating habits, the teenage years are crucial. Teens can promote their general health and well-being by making dietary improvements and improving their diets by addressing common nutritional difficulties and offering helpful techniques for overcoming them. Teenagers can create good eating habits that will last well into adulthood by addressing body image issues, encouraging regular eating patterns, promoting balanced meals, and providing nutrition education.

chapter 04
Healthy Eating on a Budget: Practical Tips for Affordable and Nutritious Meals

Although eating healthily is sometimes seen to be costly, it may actually be both inexpensive and nutrient-dense with proper preparation and decision-making. This chapter examines doable strategies for eating healthily on a tight budget, emphasizing low-cost methods of including nutrient-dense foods in regular meals. Consuming a well-balanced diet is crucial for maintaining general health and wellness, as it can aid in the prevention of chronic illnesses like obesity, diabetes, and heart disease. You can eat healthily on a tight budget without sacrificing taste or diversity by choosing wisely and giving nutrient-dense items priority. The secret to eating well on a tight budget is to organize your meals. Begin by organizing your meals for the week using recipes that are affordable and seasonal goods. To prevent impulsive purchases, create a shopping list based on your meal plan and follow it. To save time and money, think about preparing meals in bulk and freezing them.

Purchasing Wisely: When purchasing healthful foods like fruits, vegetables, whole grains, and lean proteins, keep an eye out for deals and discounts. Items with a lengthy shelf life, such grains, beans, and canned products, are best purchased in bulk. For more reasonably priced options, check out local produce stands, farmers' markets, and bargain retailers.

Selecting Foods Rich in Nutrients: Just concentrate on eating foods like fruits, vegetables, whole grains, and legumes that offer the most nutrients at the lowest cost. Think about purchasing frozen produce because it is frequently less expensive and has a longer shelf life than fresh.

Cooking in the House: In general, cooking at home is less expensive and healthier than eating out. To keep meals interesting, try out different cooking methods and recipes.
Utilize leftovers to make fresh dishes. reducing food waste and saving money.

Making Healthy Substitutions: Look for affordable alternatives to expensive ingredients. For example, use dried herbs instead of fresh, or substitute beans for meat in recipes. Consider making your own condiments and sauces to save money and reduce added sugars and preservatives.

Eating Seasonally: Seasonal produce is often more affordable and fresher than out-of-season options. Plan your meals around what's in season to save money and enjoy the best flavors. Consider growing your own herbs and vegetables to save even more money and enjoy the satisfaction of homegrown produce.

Avoiding Food Waste: Plan meals based on what you already have in your pantry and refrigerator to avoid buying unnecessary items. Use leftovers creatively to create new meals. For example, leftover vegetables can be added to soups Staying Hydrated: Water is the healthiest and most affordable beverage choice. Avoid sugary drinks and opt for water instead. Consider buying a reusable water bottle to save money and reduce waste.

Budget-Friendly Recipe Ideas: Vegetarian chili made with beans, vegetables, and spices. Lentil soup with vegetables and whole grains. Stir-fry with brown rice, mixed vegetables, and tofu or chicken. Omelets or frittatas with vegetables and whole eggs or egg whites. Pasta dishes with whole grain pasta, vegetables, and a homemade tomato sauce. Homemade pizzas with whole grain crust, vegetables, and a small amount of cheese.

Conclusion
1. Planning meals in advance and creating a shopping list can help you stick to your budget.
2. Buying seasonal fruits and vegetables can be more affordable and nutritious.
3. Purchasing store-brand or generic products can save you money without sacrificing quality.
4. Using leftovers creatively can help reduce food waste and save money.
5. Buying in bulk, especially for staple items like grains and legumes, can be cost-effective.
6. Cooking at home instead of eating out can save you money and allow you to control the ingredients in your meals.
7. Incorporating more plant-based meals into your diet can be more budget-friendly than meat-based meals.
8. Taking advantage of sales and discounts can help you save money on groceries.
9. Growing your own herbs, fruits, and vegetables can save you money and provide fresh, nutritious ingredients.
10. Prioritizing your spending on nutrient-dense foods can help you make the most of your budget and maintain a healthy diet.
Eating healthy on a budget is possible with careful planning, smart choices, and a little creativity. By focusing on nutrient-dense foods, planning meals in advance, shopping smart, and cooking at home, it is possible to enjoy delicious and nutritious meals without breaking the bank. With these practical tips, you can eat healthily, save money, and improve your overall health and well-being.

Chapter 05
Emotional Eating: Understanding the Connection Between Emotions and Food

Introduction: Emotional eating is a complex behavior that involves using food to cope with or suppress emotions. This chapter explores the connection between emotions and food, the triggers of emotional eating, and strategies to develop a healthier relationship with food.

No. Comparison Explanation

1. Nourishment Just as food nourishes the body, emotions nourish the soul, providing us with psychological sustenance.
2. Variety Both emotions and food come in a variety of forms, ranging from simple to complex.
3. Satisfaction Eating satisfying food can evoke positive emotions, such as happiness and contentment.
4. Balance Like a balanced diet, a balance of emotions is essential for overall well-being.
5. Impact on Health Unhealthy food choices can negatively impact physical health, while negative emotions can affect mental health.
6. Social Connection Food often brings people together, fostering social connections, much like emotions do.
7. Cultural Significance Both food and emotions can hold significant cultural meaning and play a role in traditions.
8. Comfort foods are often associated with feelings of warmth and comfort, much like comforting emotions.
9. Seasonal Influence Both food preferences and emotional states can be influenced by the seasons.
10. Indulgence Indulging in certain foods or emotions can provide temporary pleasure or relief.

11. Psychological Response Food and emotions can both elicit strong psychological responses, such as cravings or nostalgia.
12. Regulation Like food, emotions need to be regulated to maintain emotional balance and prevent excess.
13. Sensory Experience Both food and emotions can provide rich sensory experiences, such as taste, smell, and touch.
14. Influence on Behavior Both food choices and emotional states can influence our behavior and decision-making.
15. Memory Recall Certain foods and emotions can trigger vivid memories from the past.
16. Coping Mechanism Some people use food as a coping mechanism for dealing with emotions, known as emotional eating.
17. Energy Source Food is a source of physical energy, while emotions can provide mental and emotional energy.
18. Satisfaction vs. Satiety While food provides satiety, emotions can provide a sense of satisfaction or fulfillment.
19. Reward System Both food and emotions can activate the brain's reward system, leading to feelings of pleasure.
20. Personal Relationship The relationship we have with food and with our emotions can be deeply personal and unique.

Understanding Emotional Eating: Emotional eating is a coping mechanism used to manage emotions such as stress, boredom, sadness, or loneliness. It involves eating in response to emotions rather than physical hunger, often leading to overeating and feelings of guilt or shame. Common Triggers of **Emotional Eating: Stress:** Stress can trigger emotional eating as a way to seek comfort or distraction from stressful situations. Boredom: Boredom can lead to mindless eating as a way to fill time or entertain oneself. Sadness: Sadness can trigger emotional eating as a way to numb or mask feelings of sadness. Loneliness: Feelings of loneliness can lead to emotional eating as a way to seek comfort and companionship. The Impact of Emotional Eating on Health: Emotional eating can lead to weight gain and obesity, as well as a range of health problems such as heart disease, diabetes, and depression. It can also contribute to a cycle of guilt, shame, and further emotional eating, creating a negative relationship with food.

Developing Awareness of Emotional Eating: One of the first steps in addressing emotional eating is developing awareness of when and why it occurs. Keeping a food diary can help identify patterns of emotional eating and the emotions that trigger it. Strategies to Overcome Emotional Eating: Identify Triggers: Become aware of the emotions and situations that trigger emotional eating. Find Alternative Coping Mechanisms: Develop healthy ways to cope with emotions, such as exercise, meditation, or talking to a friend. Practice Mindful Eating: Pay attention to your hunger cues and eat slowly to fully enjoy and appreciate your food. Keep Healthy Foods on Hand: Stock your kitchen with healthy, satisfying foods to reduce the temptation of unhealthy snacks. Seek Support: Talk to a therapist or counselor if
emotional eating is a persistent issue that you struggle to manage on your own. Cognitive Behavioral Therapy (CBT) for Emotional Eating: CBT can help individuals identify and change the negative thought patterns and behaviors that contribute to emotional eating.

Mindfulness-Based Eating Practices: Mindfulness practices, such as mindful eating, can help individuals become more aware of their eating habits and the emotions driving them. By practicing mindfulness, individuals can learn to eat more intuitively and break free from emotional eating patterns. Creating a Healthy Relationship with Food: Developing a healthy relationship with food involves viewing food as nourishment for the body rather than a source of comfort or punishment. It also involves practicing self-compassion and forgiveness when it comes to food choices.

Conclusion: Emotional eating is a common behavior that can have negative impacts on physical and emotional health. By developing awareness of emotional eating triggers and practicing healthy coping mechanisms, individuals can develop a healthier relationship with food and improve overall well-being.

chapter 06
Body Image and Nutrition: How Body Image Influences Eating Habits

Introduction

Body image plays a significant role in shaping our relationship with food and eating habits. This chapter explores the complex relationship between body image and nutrition, the impact of body image on eating behaviors, and strategies to foster a positive body image and healthy eating habits.

Understanding Body Image: Body image refers to how we perceive, think about, and feel about our bodies. It is influenced by a variety of factors, including cultural ideals, media representation, social comparisons, and personal experiences. The Impact of Body Image on Eating Habits: Negative body image can lead to disordered eating behaviors, such as restrictive dieting, binge eating, or compulsive exercising. Conversely, a positive body image is associated with healthier eating habits and a more balanced approach to Media Influence on Body Image: Media, including magazines, television, and social media, often promote unrealistic body ideals that can contribute to negative body image. Constant exposure to these ideals can lead to dissatisfaction with one's own body and unhealthy eating behaviors. **Cultural and Social Influences on Body Image:** Cultural ideals of beauty vary widely and can impact how individuals perceive their own bodies. Social comparisons with peers or celebrities can also influence body image and eating behaviors. Eating Disorders and Body Image: Eating disorders, such as anorexia nervosa, bulimia nervosa, and binge eating disorder, are often characterized by distorted body image and unhealthy eating habits. These disorders can have serious physical and psychological consequences and require professional treatment.

Strategies for Fostering a Positive Body Image: Practice Self-Compassion: Be kind and compassionate towards yourself, and avoid self-criticism based on body image. Focus on Health, Not Weight: Shift the focus from weight and appearance to overall health and well-being. Surround Yourself with Positive Influences: Surround yourself with people who support and uplift you, and limit exposure to negative body image messages in the media. Practice Mindful Eating: Eat slowly, savoring each bite, and pay attention to hunger and fullness cues. Seek Professional Help: If body image issues are impacting your mental or physical health, consider seeking support from a therapist or counselor.

Promoting Positive Body Image in Children and Adolescents: Encourage Healthful Behaviors: Focus on healthful behaviors rather than appearance, such as being active and eating a balanced diet. Be a Positive Role Model: Model positive body image and healthy eating habits for children and adolescents. Teach Media Literacy: Teach children and adolescents to critically evaluate media messages about body image and beauty. Conclusion: Body image plays a significant role in shaping our relationship with food and eating habits. By fostering a positive body image and promoting healthy eating behaviors, individuals can improve their overall well-being and quality of life.

chapter 07
Eating Disorders: Recognizing the Signs and Seeking Help

Introduction
Eating Disorder Sign/Action Description
1. Dramatic weight loss or gain Significant changes in weight that are not due to intentional dieting or exercise.
2. Obsession with body weight and shape Constantly talking about weight, body image, and dissatisfaction with appearance.
3. Preoccupation with food and calories Excessive focus on calorie counting, food preparation, and avoiding certain food groups.
4. Eating in secret or hoarding food Hiding food, eating alone, or hoarding food in unusual places.
5. Excessive exercise Working out excessively, even when injured or exhausted, and feeling guilty when unable to exercise.
6. Avoidance of social gatherings involving food Avoiding social events that involve food or making excuses to avoid eating in public.
7. Mood swings and irritability Sudden changes in mood, including depression, anxiety, or irritability.
8. Physical signs such as dizziness or fainting Experiencing dizziness, fainting, or weakness due to inadequate nutrition.
9. Dental issues such as tooth decay Tooth decay or discoloration from repeated vomiting or excessive consumption of sugary foods.
10. Changes in eating habits Skipping meals, following strict diets, or adopting unusual eating rituals.
11. Wearing baggy clothes to hide body shape Wearing loose-fitting clothing to hide weight loss or gain. 12.

Expressing feelings of guilt or shame Feeling guilty or ashamed about eating habits or body shape.
13. Difficulty concentrating or focusing Experiencing trouble concentrating or focusing on tasks due to lack of nutrition.
14. Social withdrawal Withdrawing from social activities or relationships due to concerns about body image.
15. Using laxatives or diuretics Using laxatives or diuretics to control weight or reduce bloating.
16. Change in menstrual cycle Irregular periods or the absence of menstruation (amenorrhea) in females.
17. Seeking isolation during or after meals Eating alone, avoiding eating with others, or isolating oneself after meals.
18. Frequent trips to the bathroom after meals Making frequent trips to the bathroom after meals, possibly to purge.
19. Denial of eating disorder behaviors Denying or minimizing concerns about eating habits, weight, or body image.
20. Seeking help from a healthcare professional Recognizing the signs of an eating disorder and seeking help from a doctor or therapist.

Eating disorders are serious mental health conditions characterized by abnormal eating habits that can have severe physical and emotional consequences. This chapter explores the different types of eating disorders, their causes, signs, and symptoms, as well as the importance of seeking help for those affected. Understanding Eating Disorders: Eating disorders are complex conditions that involve a range of psychological, biological, and environmental factors. They are not just about food, but also about feelings of control, self-worth, and body image.

Types of Eating Disorders

Anorexia Nervosa: Characterized by extreme restriction of food intake, fear of gaining weight, and a distorted body image. **Bulimia Nervosa**: Characterized by episodes of binge eating followed by purging behaviors, such as vomiting or excessive exercise. **Disorder Binge Eating**: Characterized by recurrent episodes of binge eating without purging behaviors.

Causes of Eating Disorders

Genetics: There is evidence to suggest that genetics play a role in the development of eating disorders. **Psychological Factors**: Low self-esteem, perfectionism, and body dissatisfaction are common psychological factors associated with eating disorders. Sociocultural Factors: Societal pressures to be thin, as well as media images portraying unrealistic body ideals, can contribute to the development of eating disorders.

Signs and Symptoms of Eating Disorders

Dramatic weight loss or gain. Obsession with food, calories, and weight. Preoccupation with body image and appearance. Extreme mood swings and changes in behavior. Avoidance of social situations involving food.

Health Consequences of Eating Disorders: Eating disorders can have serious physical consequences, including: Malnutrition Dehydration Electrolyte imbalances Heart problems Digestive issues Bone loss They can also have severe emotional and psychological effects, including depression, anxiety, and social isolation. Getting Help for Eating Disorders: Recognizing the signs and symptoms of an eating disorder is the first step to getting help. Treatment typically involves a combination of therapy, nutritional counseling, and medical monitoring. Family therapy may also be beneficial, especially for adolescents with eating

disorders. Recovery from Eating Disorders: Recovery from
an eating disorder is possible with the right treatment and support. It is important for individuals in recovery to develop a healthy relationship with food and their bodies. Recovery is a journey, and it may involve setbacks, but with perseverance and support, individuals can regain control of their health and well-being.

Keeping Eating Disorders at Bay:
Teaching youth about appropriate eating practices, body image, and self-esteem can help avert eating disorders. It can also be advantageous to support body positivity and a positive connection with eating.

In summary:
Treatment from a specialist is necessary for eating disorders, which are major mental health issues.

The first steps in recovery include identifying the warning signs and symptoms of an eating disorder and getting help as soon as possible.

People with eating disorders can recover and lead healthy, meaningful lives with the correct care and assistance.

Chapter 08
Balanced Eating for Busy Teens: Strategies for Eating Well with a Busy Schedule

First of all,

Teenage years are frequently characterized by hectic schedules that include extracurricular activities, school, social engagements, and other things. Teens should emphasize their diet and health in spite of these obligations. This chapter examines balanced eating tactics for teenagers who lead busy lives, emphasizing useful advice to support them in keeping a nutritious diet in spite of their demanding schedules.

Recognizing the Value of a Balanced Diet

Teenage growth and development require a balanced diet since it provides the nutrients required for energy, cognitive function, and general health. Eating a balanced diet can boost a teen's immune system, help them maintain a healthy weight, and lower their chance of developing chronic illnesses in the future.

Problems of a Busy Schedule with Eating well

Time Restrictions: It can be challenging to find time due to hectic schedules. to cook and consume wholesome food. Availability of Healthy Options: Choosing healthfully can be difficult if there are few healthy food options available, such as fast food or convenience store snacks.

Peer Influence: Unhealthy eating habits can result from peer pressure and social influences on food choices.

Plan Ahead: Give yourself enough time to organize your weekly menu, taking into account your schedule and the availability of wholesome options.

Plan your meals ahead of time: Make a lot of food in advance and portion it out into freezer-safe pieces for quick and simple meals all week long.
Carry Nuts, Fruits, and Yogurt as Healthy Snacks: To steer clear of unhealthy vending machine selections, always have nuts, fruits, and vegetables on hand as healthy snacks.
Select Healthful Fast Food Options: When dining out, stay away from fried foods and opt instead for salads, grilled chicken sandwiches, or wraps.
Keep Yourself Hydrated: Avoid sugar-filled drinks and stay hydrated by drinking lots of water throughout the day.

Ideas for a Balanced Lunch and Snack:
Breakfast consists of whole grain toast with avocado, Greek yogurt with granola and berries, and eggs scrambled or a spinach, banana, and protein powder smoothie. Lunch options include quinoa salad with veggies and chickpeas, tuna sandwich on whole grain toast, or a turkey and cheese whole grain wrap.
Dinner options include lean ground turkey, whole grain spaghetti with marinara sauce, and grilled chicken served with quinoa or mixed veggies and tofu stir-fried over brown rice.
Snacks: whole grain crackers with cheese, bananas with nut butter, hummus and vegetable sticks, or Greek yogurt with berries.
Conscious Eating Techniques
To avoid overindulging and facilitate better digestion, take your time eating and enjoy every bite.
To minimize mindless eating and to concentrate on your food, avoid dining in front of screens, such as a TV

or computer. Observe your body's hunger signals and cease Eating should occur when you're satisfied but not full.

Including Physical Activity in a Busy Schedule:

Teenagers should engage in regular physical activity as part of a healthy lifestyle.

Find ways to stay active during the day, such as biking or walking to school, using the stairs rather than the elevator, or engaging in extracurricular sports or activities.

Creating Lifelong Healthy Habits:

Involve teens in meal planning and preparation to help them take charge of their nutrition and overall health. Instruct them on the value of moderation and balance, as well as how to make good decisions in any circumstance.

In conclusion, it is feasible to prioritize your health and eat well even with a busy schedule.

Teenagers that implement these techniques into their daily lives can keep a balanced even with a busy schedule, maintain their general health and well-being through eating.

Chapter 9
How to Meet Your Nutritional Needs Without Eating Meat or Using Animal Products

First of all,
Diets that are vegetarian or vegan have become more and more popular in recent years because of their possible health advantages and moral implications. Meat and, in the case of veganism, all animal products are off limits in these diets. The nutritional characteristics of vegetarian and vegan diets are examined in this chapter, along with suggestions for embracing a vegetarian or vegan lifestyle, potential health benefits, and how to meet nutrient demands.

Comprehending Vegan and Vegetarian Diets:
Meat is not a part of a vegetarian diet, although dairy and eggs may be.
A vegan diet consists of avoiding any animal products, such as dairy, eggs, meat, and honey.

Nutrition-Related Considerations
Protein: Legumes, tofu, tempeh, seitan, nuts, seeds, and whole grains are plant-based sources of protein. To guarantee that you are getting enough of the essential amino acids, mix and match different sources of protein throughout the day.
Iron: Legumes, beans, tofu, spinach, and fortified cereals are plant-based sources of iron. Iron absorption can be improved by eating foods high in vitamin C, such as bell peppers and citrus fruits.
Calcium: Fortified plant milks, tofu, leafy green vegetables, almonds, and sesame seeds are among the plant-based sources of calcium. The absorption of calcium also depends on a sufficient intake of vitamin D.
Vitamin B12: Animal sources are the main source of vitamin B12. products, so in order to guarantee proper

intake, vegans should incorporate foods or supplements that have been fortified.

Fatty acids omega-3: Omega-3 fatty acids can be obtained from plants by eating flaxseeds, chia seeds, hemp seeds, walnuts, and supplements made of algae.

The health advantages of vegan and vegetarian diets

Decreased risk of chronic illnesses: Studies have linked vegan and vegetarian diets to a lower risk of heart disease, high blood pressure, type 2 diabetes, and several cancers.

Weight control: Diets based mostly on plants tend to be lower in calories and saturated fat, which may help with weight control.

Better digestion: Diets based mostly on plants tend to have more fiber, which can help to maintain regular bowel motions and gut health.

Possible Aspects for Health

Deficiencies in some nutrients: Vegans and vegetarians may be susceptible to low levels of iron, calcium, vitamin B12, and omega-3 fatty acids, in particular. Meal planning is crucial, and if needed, supplements should be taken into account.

Protein quality: While plant-based proteins may not include as many important amino acids as animal proteins, consuming a variety of plant-based protein sources will help guarantee sufficient consumption.

Advice on Changing to a Vegan or Vegetarian Diet

Begin cautiously: Reduce your meat intake gradually and try new plant-based recipes and meals.

Become knowledgeable: Find out how to meet the nutritional needs of a plant-based diet and the requirements of a vegetarian or vegan diet.

Arrange your meals: To guarantee sufficient nutritional intake, prepare meals that are balanced and incorporate a range of plant-based foods.

Think about supplements: See your doctor if you require any supplements for calcium, iron, vitamin B12, or omega-3 fatty acids.

Overcoming Practical and Social Obstacles:
When dining out, seek for establishments that cater to vegetarians or vegans, or select recipes that are easily adaptable to fit with these diets.

Families and social events: Let others know what you eat or don't eat, and offer to bring a food to share.

When traveling, look for eateries that cater to vegetarians or vegans and bring meals or snacks.

No. Final Thought
1. Diets based solely on plants can supply all the nutrients required for general health.
2. Plant-based foods like beans, lentils, tofu, and tempeh can help vegetarians and vegans acquire the protein they need.
3. Plant-based sources of iron include spinach, lentils, and fortified cereals; however, consuming these meals in combination with foods high in vitamin C can improve absorption.
4. In addition to kale and broccoli, fortified plant milks and tofu also contain calcium.
5. You may get omega-3 fatty acids from walnuts, chia seeds, and flaxseeds. These fatty acids are vital for heart health and cognitive function.
6. Because vitamin B12 is mostly found in animal sources, it should be supplemented in a plant-based diet as it is necessary for nerve function and the generation of red blood cells.
7. Legumes, nuts, seeds, and whole grains are good sources of zinc, which is necessary for both immunological response and wound healing.

8. itamin D is essential for healthy bones and can be acquired from sun exposure, mushrooms, and plant milks that have been fortified.

9. The secret to ensuring that a plant-based diet meets all nutritional demands is meticulous meal planning that incorporates a range of foods.

10. Speaking with a doctor or nutritionist can assist guarantee that a plant-based diet is individualized and fits nutritional needs.

chapter 10
Nutrition for Athletic Performance: Fueling the Body for Sports and Physical Activity

First of all,

Athlete performance is greatly impacted by nutrition, which supplies the energy and nutrients required to power exercises, aid in recuperation, and improve general performance. The main ideas of nutrition for sports performance are covered in this chapter, along with the functions of micronutrients, macronutrients, hydration, and supplements.

Recognizing Energy Requirements:

Calorie-wise, energy comes from the food we eat, mostly from proteins, lipids, and carbohydrates.

Because they burn more energy and have more muscle mass than sedentary people, athletes need more calories.

The Role of Macronutrients in Sports Performance

Carbohydrates: For athletes, especially during high-intensity exercise, carbohydrates are the main energy source. Whole grains, fruits, vegetables, and legumes are good sources.

Proteins: Building and repairing muscle requires proteins. Athletes should eat enough protein from various sources. such as fish, poultry, dairy products, lentils, lean meats, and plant-based protein sources.

Fats: Essential for the synthesis of hormones and the integrity of cell membranes, fats are a concentrated form of energy. Olive oil, almonds, seeds, and avocados are good sources of healthy fats.

The Role of Micronutrients in Sports Performance

Minerals and vitamins are essential for the synthesis of energy, the health of muscles, and recuperation. To make sure they obtain an adequate intake of micronutrients, athletes should eat a range of fruits, vegetables, whole grains, and lean meats. Because they support fluid balance and muscular function, electrolytes like sodium, potassium, and magnesium are especially crucial for athletes who perform extended or vigorous activity.

Hydration in Sports

Drinking enough water is crucial for optimal sports performance. Before, during, and after exercise, athletes should consume lots of fluids to replenish lost fluids and electrolytes.

While sports drinks with electrolytes may be helpful for intense or extended activity, water is usually adequate for hydration during moderate exercise.
Meal timing and composition:

To guarantee they have enough energy to execute, athletes should have a balanced breakfast with carbohydrates, proteins, and fats two to three hours before exercising.

To get a quick energy boost, have a modest snack with protein and carbs 30 to 60 minutes before working out. Athletes should have a meal or snack high in protein and carbs after working out to aid in muscle repair and glycogen replenishment.

Supplementing to Boost Athletic Performance: As a While most athletes can get all the nutrients they require from a well-balanced diet, some may find that supplements are helpful.

Branched-chain amino acids, creatine, beta-alanine, and protein powders are common supplements taken by athletes (BCAAs). It's crucial to speak with a healthcare professional before beginning any supplements program.

Organizing Meals for Athletes:
Athletes must to concentrate on eating foods high in nutrients and with a sensible ratio of fats, proteins, and carbs.

Athletes may support their training and performance goals by ensuring they get the nutrients they need by planning meals and snacks in advance.

Particular Things to Think About for Endurance Athletes

Because endurance athletes engage in prolonged physical activity, such as marathon runners and bikers, their needs for carbohydrates may be higher. To keep their energy levels stable, these athletes should concentrate on eating enough carbs before, during, and after exercise.

No. Point of Conclusion

1. For athletes to compete at their peak and recover quickly, they must eat a healthy diet.
2. A substantial amount of an athlete's diet should consist of carbohydrates as they are their main fuel source.
3. Athletes should strive to incorporate high-quality protein sources into their diets because proteins are essential for both muscle building and repair.
4. Athletes should also consume fats, but in moderation, as they maintain general health and provide energy.
5. Drinking enough of fluids before, during, and after exercise is essential for athletes to function at their best.
6. Sweating causes the loss of electrolytes like sodium and potassium, which should be replaced both before and after exercise, particularly in hot weather.
7. It's crucial to schedule meals and snacks around exercise sessions in order to help recuperation afterward and supply energy when it's most needed.

8. Timing your nutrition intake, such as eating protein and carbohydrates soon after working out, helps improve muscle repair and recovery.

9. Certain athletes may benefit from supplements, but they should be used cautiously and under the supervision of a medical professional or sports nutritionist.

10. Customized diet programs are essential for maximizing sports performance; players should consult a nutritionist to create a plan that meets their unique needs.

chapter 11
Mindful Eating: Techniques for Eating with Awareness and Enjoyment

First of all,

The practice of mindful eating entails giving your undivided attention to the entire eating experience, including the food and any physical reactions that may occur. The foundations of mindful eating, its advantages, and doable methods for implementing mindful eating into your everyday life are all covered in this chapter.

Comprehending Intentional Eating:

No. Information on Topic

1. Definition The discipline of being completely present and cognizant of the dining experience is known as mindful eating.
2. Mindful Eating It entails observing the tastes, textures, aromas, colors, and experiences of food.
3. Deceleration Eating mindfully promotes taking your time, enjoying each bite, and eating slowly.
4. Listening to Hunger Cues In order to choose when and how much to eat, one must pay attention to the body's signals of hunger and fullness.
5. Empathy-Based Observation Practitioners observe, without condemnation or critique, their feelings and thoughts toward eating.
6. Accepting the Situation non-reactive awareness of food, eating, and the body's cues is promoted by mindful eating.
7. Recognizing Emotional Consumption It enables people to distinguish between physical hunger and hunger for emotions.
8. Fostering Appreciation A spirit of thankfulness for the food, the company, and the surroundings is fostered by mindful eating.

9. Enhanced Digestion Eating with awareness helps the body absorb and process nutrients more efficiently, which in turn helps with digestion.

10. Encouraging Nutritious Food Practices It can result in less overeating, healthier food selections, and a more positive

The Buddhist idea of mindfulness, which entails being totally present and aware in the moment, is the foundation of mindful eating. It entails observing your food's hues, scents, tastes, textures, and temperatures in addition to your body's feelings of hunger and fullness. Mindful eating is about creating a healthy and balanced relationship with food, not about dieting or limiting one's intake.

Advantages of Intentional Eating:

Enhanced meal enjoyment: You can savor and appreciate your food to the fullest by focusing on the sensory aspects of eating.

Better digestion: Eating mindfully can make you more conscious of your body's signals of hunger and fullness, which will help you prepare meals that are more satisfying and well-balanced.

Managing weight: By consuming more food If you eat slowly and deliberately, you might be more aware of your body's natural hunger and fullness cues and less prone to overindulge.

Decreased emotional eating: By practicing mindful eating, you can learn better coping skills and become more conscious of the emotional triggers that cause overeating.

The fundamentals of mindful eating

Eating mindfully and slowly: Take your time, enjoy each bite, and avoid eating in front of the phone, computer, or TV.

Observing signs of hunger and fullness Even if there is food left on your plate, you should only eat until you are satisfied.

Observing how food affects your body: Be aware of the physical and mental effects that certain foods have on you.

Using every sense possible: Take note of your food's hues, flavors, textures, aromas, and temperatures.

Methods for Putting Mindful Eating into Practice:
Prior to eating, take a few minutes to sit still and concentrate on your breathing while practicing mindful eating meditation. Without passing judgment, take note of any thoughts or feelings that surface.

Exercises for mindful eating: Take a tiny bit of food, such a slice of apple or a raisin, and carefully inspect it before consuming it slowly and relishing every taste.

Eating mindfully in daily life: When you eat, concentrate on taking your time and enjoying every bite of your food. Aim to focus on the flavors and textures of your food rather than becoming distracted.

Some Advice for Including Mindful Eating in Your Everyday Life

Start modest: Start with one meal or snack per day to start practicing mindful eating, and as it becomes more comfortable, progressively increase the frequency.

Be patient with yourself and approach mindful eating with an open mind and curiosity because it is a skill that takes time to master.

Engage in self-compassion: If you see yourself getting irritated or critical throughout your practice, tell yourself it's acceptable to experience these emotions and gently bring your attention back to the here and now.

Conscious Eating and Losing Weight:
Although mindful eating is not a diet, it can support a more balanced and aware relationship with food, which makes it a useful tool for managing weight. Eating thoughtfully can help you develop more enduring and healthier eating habits by reducing your tendency to overeat and improving your awareness of your body's signals of hunger and fullness.

In summary
It's possible to have a healthier and more fulfilling relationship with food by practicing mindful eating. You may enhance your digestion, increase your awareness of your body's hunger and fullness signals, and savor and appreciate your meal to the fullest by adopting mindful eating practices into your daily life.

chapter 12
Food and Mood: How Diet Affects Mental Health and Well-being

First of all,
Food and mood have a complicated and multidimensional interaction. Diet has a significant impact on mood, cognition, and brain function overall, which is important for mental health and wellbeing. This chapter examines the relationship between nutrition and mental health, the function of particular nutrients in mood regulation, and helpful dietary maintenance advice.

The Brain-Gut Relationship:
The gut and the brain communicate with each other in both directions through the gut-brain axis.
This communication is mediated by the gut microbiome, which affects behavior, mood, and brain function.

Dietary Influence on Mental Health:
High intake of processed foods, sugar, and harmful fats characterizes a poor diet, which is linked to a higher risk of mental health conditions including depression. and unease.
On the other hand, a diet high in fruits, vegetables, whole grains, lean meats, and healthy fats is linked to better mood and a decreased risk of mental health issues.

Essential Minerals for Mental Wellness:
Omega-3 fatty acids: Essential for brain function and mood modulation, omega-3 fatty acids can be found in walnuts, flaxseeds, and fatty fish.

B vitamins: B vitamins, especially folate, B6, and B12, are essential for the production of neurotransmitters and the control of mood. They can be found in meals including meat, eggs, beans, and leafy green vegetables.

Magnesium: The body uses magnesium for approximately 300 metabolic processes, some of which are connected to mood control. Nuts, seeds, whole grains, and leafy green vegetables are among the foods that contain it.

Zinc: Zinc is necessary for both mood modulation and brain function. Foods including oysters, poultry, red meat, beans, and nuts contain it.

Antioxidants: Vitamins C and E are examples of antioxidants that help shield the brain from oxidative damage.

Omega-3 fatty acids: Essential for brain function and mood modulation, omega-3 fatty acids can be found in walnuts, flaxseeds, and fatty fish.

B vitamins: B vitamins, especially folate, B6, and B12, are essential for the production of neurotransmitters and the control of mood. They can be found in meals including meat, eggs, beans, and leafy green vegetables.

Magnesium: The body uses magnesium for approximately 300 metabolic processes, some of which are connected to mood control. Nuts, seeds, whole grains, and leafy green vegetables are among the foods that contain it.

Zinc: Zinc is necessary for both mood modulation and brain function. Foods including oysters, poultry, red meat, beans, and nuts contain it.

Antioxidants: Vitamins C and E are examples of antioxidants that help shield the brain from oxidative damage. inflammation and stress. Nuts, seeds, fruits, and vegetables all contain them.

Sugar's and processed foods' roles:
An elevated risk of anxiety and depression is linked to high consumption of processed foods and sugar.
Blood sugar swings brought on by these foods may have an adverse effect on mood and energy levels.

Tips for Mindful Eating to Lift Your Mood:
Consume food mindfully, taking time to appreciate its flavors, textures, and sensory qualities with each bite.
To ensure that you are completely focused on your meal, avoid any distractions like watching TV or using electronics while you are eating.
Pay attention to your body's signals of hunger and fullness to know when to eat and when to quit.
Remind yourself to be grateful for the food you eat and the health benefits it offers your body and mind.

Hydration's Effect on Mood:
Fatigue, irritability, and lack of focus are all symptoms of dehydration that can have a detrimental effect on mood.
To maintain proper brain function and stay hydrated, make it a point to sip on lots of water throughout the day.

Including Foods That Improve Mood in Your Diet:
Omega-3 fatty acid-rich fatty fish: fatty fish such To maintain proper brain function and stay hydrated, make it a point to sip on lots of water throughout the day.

Including Foods That Improve Mood in Your Diet
Fatty fish: Packed with omega-3 fatty acids, fatty fish like sardines, mackerel, and salmon can promote mood management and brain health.
Leafy green vegetables: Rich in antioxidants, vitamins, and minerals, leafy greens like Swiss chard, spinach, and kale can help shield the brain and elevate mood.
Berries: Packed with vitamins and antioxidants, berries are an excellent option for promoting mental and emotional well-being.
Nuts and seeds: Rich in magnesium, zinc, and good fats, nuts and seeds are essential for brain function and mood management.
Useful Hints for Including Foods that Boost Mood:

To provide a wide spectrum of nutrients, including a variety of fruits and vegetables in your diet, striving for varied colors.

Select whole grains over refined grains to help maintain stable mood and blood sugar levels.

Include plant-based protein sources in your diet, such as lentils, beans, tofu, and tempeh.

Eat less processed food, sweetened drinks, and unhealthy fats as these can have a detrimental effect on your mood.

Point of Conclusion

1. Because diet affects mood, thought, and behavior, it is important for mental health and well-being.
2. Better mental health outcomes are linked to eating a diet high in fruits, vegetables, whole grains, and lean meats.
3. Deficiencies in certain nutrients, such iron, B vitamins, and omega-3 fatty acids, can have a detrimental impact on mental and emotional well-being.
4. Consuming unhealthy fats, sweets, and processed meals in excess is associated with a higher risk of anxiety and sadness.
5. The gut microbiome affects mood and brain function, and the gut-brain axis is important for mental health.
6. Mood swings, irritation, and exhaustion may be attributed to blood sugar variations resulting from a high-sugar diet.
7. Even mild dehydration can impair cognitive function, thus maintaining proper hydration is crucial for brain health and mood management.
8. Mindful eating techniques, such savoring food and observing hunger cues, can enhance mood and foster a good relationship with food.

9. Individual variations in the relationship between food and mood emphasize the significance of tailored dietary strategies for mental well-being.

10. In general, consuming a diet high in nutrients and balance is key to supporting mental health and well-being.

Diet has a big impact on mental health and wellbeing since it affects emotion, thinking, and brain function in general.

You may foster optimal mental health and enhance your general well-being by increasing your intake of nutrient-rich foods and engaging in mindful eating.

chapter 13
Nutritional Supplements: Understanding When and How to Use Supplements Safely

First of all,

Products known as nutritional supplements are made to offer nutrients to those who might not get enough of them from their usual diet. Supplements are not a substitute for a balanced diet, even though they may help certain people. The use of nutritional supplements is examined in this chapter, along with situations in which they might be advantageous, safe usage guidelines, and concerns for certain populations.

Comprehending Nutritional Supplements:

There are many different types of nutritional supplements, such as vitamins, minerals, herbal remedies, enzymes, and amino acids. They shouldn't be used in place of a balanced diet; rather, they are meant to be a supplement.

When Supplements Could Be Helpful

Nutrient shortages: People with recognized nutrient shortages, such as a vitamin D deficit, may benefit from taking supplements.

Quality: Select dietary supplements from reliable companies that follow quality guidelines and have undergone purity and potency testing.

Dosage: Unless a healthcare professional advises you differently, adhere to the suggested dosage guidelines listed on the supplement package.

Interactions: Before beginning a new supplement regimen, it's crucial to speak with a healthcare professional as some supplements may interact with other supplements or drugs.

Side Effects: If you have any negative responses, stop using the supplement. You should be aware of the possible side effects of supplements.

Frequently Used Dietary Supplements:
Vitamin D: Essential for immunological response, mood control, and bone health. Supplementing may be beneficial for a large number of people, particularly those who live in northern latitudes or receive little sun exposure.
Omega-3 Fatty Acids: Crucial for heart and brain function as well as the management of inflammation. Located in fatty fish and supplements made of algae.
Probiotics: Good microorganisms that aid with digestion and intestinal health. found in dietary supplements and fermented foods.
Calcium: necessary for strong bones. most frequently seen in vitamins and dairy products.
Iron: Essential for the production of red blood cells and the movement of oxygen. Iron deficiency is prevalent, particularly in vegetarians and women of reproductive age.

How to Safely Use Supplements

Before beginning any new supplement regimen, especially if you have underlying medical concerns or are taking medication, speak with your healthcare professional.
Select dietary supplements from reliable companies that have undergone quality and purity testing.
Observe the suggested dosage guidelines provided on the supplement label.
Recognize any possible conflicts with prescription drugs or other dietary supplements.
Keep an eye out for any adverse effects and stop using if required.
In summary: For certain people, nutritional supplements may be helpful, particularly if they have

higher dietary requirements or certain vitamin shortages.

It's crucial to use supplements responsibly, to adhere to dose guidelines, and to see a doctor before beginning a new supplement program.

Recall that a balanced diet is still preferable to taking supplements, so concentrate on getting your nutrients from food.

Final Thought

1. People with certain medical illnesses or dietary inadequacies may benefit from nutritional supplements.
2. Before beginning any new supplement regimen, it's crucial to speak with a healthcare professional, particularly if you have underlying medical conditions or are taking medication.
3. Supplements should be used to fill in nutrient gaps rather than as a substitute for a balanced diet.
4. Knowing your specific nutritional requirements through dietary analysis or blood testing will assist you in determining whether or not you need to take any supplements.
5. Selecting premium supplements from reliable manufacturers can assist guarantee their efficacy and safety.
6. Pay attention to the suggested dosage guidelines when using supplements, as exceeding them can have negative effects.
7. Exercise caution when using supplements that Excessive claims or promises of quick remedies should be avoided since they might not be backed up by scientific data.
8. A balanced diet and frequent exercise are already components of a healthy lifestyle; supplements should be used to support these aspects of it.

9. Some groups of people should speak with a healthcare professional since they may require different supplements than others, including the elderly, children, and pregnant women.

10. Keep an eye out for any possible interactions between your prescription drugs and supplements, since certain supplements may reduce the efficacy of your meds.

11. When you start a new supplement, note any adverse effects or changes in your health and talk to your doctor about them.

12. Properly store supplements out of children's reach and away from sunlight in a cool, dry location.

13. Should you encounter If you have any negative side effects from a supplement, stop taking it right once and see a doctor.

14. Check in with your healthcare practitioner on a regular basis to make sure your supplement regimen is still appropriate for your needs.

15. To sum up, although supplements may be helpful in some circumstances, it's critical to utilize them cautiously and under a doctor's supervision.

chapter 14
Eating for Healthy Skin: Foods that Promote Clear, Healthy Skin

In addition to reflecting good external skincare habits, good nutrition and interior wellness also contribute to healthy skin. Our skin's appearance and health can be significantly influenced by the foods we eat. The significance of diet in producing clear, healthy skin is examined in this chapter, along with the greatest foods for skin health, nutrients that promote skin function, and dietary advice for keeping skin glowing.

Recognizing the Impact of Nutrition on Skin Health:
The biggest organ in the body, the skin acts as a barrier to protect the body from the elements.
Because diet provides vital nutrients that support skin function and regeneration, it can have an impact on skin health.

Top Foods for Skin Health:
Omega-3 fatty acids are abundant in fatty fish, which includes mackerel, salmon, and Sardines are a good way to keep skin hydrated and prevent inflammation.
Avocados: Packed full of antioxidants, healthy fats, and vitamins C and E, avocados can help hydrate and protect skin.
Nuts and Seeds: Packed with of vitamins, minerals, and good fats, nuts and seeds can help keep skin looking young and stave off aging symptoms.
Leafy Greens: Vitamins A, C, and E are essential for skin health and healing and are abundant in kale, spinach, and other leafy greens.
Berries: Rich in antioxidants, berries can help shield the skin from oxidative damage brought on by free radicals.

Sweet potatoes: Packed in beta-carotene, sweet potatoes can shield the skin from UV ray damage and enhance the general health of the skin.

The Right Nutrients for Good Skin

Antioxidant vitamin C: Aids in preserving the Vitamin C, which protects skin from harm, can be found in bell peppers, strawberries, and citrus fruits.

Vitamin E: Found in nuts, seeds, and spinach, vitamin E is another antioxidant that aids in shielding the skin from harm.

Vitamin A: Found in liver, carrots, and sweet potatoes, vitamin A is essential for skin upkeep and repair.

Omega-3 Fatty Acids: Flaxseeds, walnuts, and fatty fish are good sources of these acids, which also assist to keep skin hydrated and prevent inflammation.

Zinc: Found in meat, seafood, and legumes, zinc is essential for wound healing and skin integrity maintenance.

Nutritional Advice for Skin Health

Keep Yourself Hydrated: To keep your skin hydrated and help remove toxins, sip lots of water throughout the day.

Limit Sugar and Processed Foods: Consuming excessive amounts of sugar and processed foods might lead to skin problems and irritation. Instead, choose complete, nutrient-dense foods.

Incorporate Foods High in Antioxidants: Leafy greens, berries, nuts, and seeds are high in antioxidants that can help shield the skin from harm.

Consume a Healthy Diet: The nutrients required for healthy skin can be obtained from a diet high in whole grains, lean meats, fruits, vegetables, and healthy fats.

Items to Steer Clear of for Good Skin

Sugar: Consuming too much sugar can aggravate skin conditions and cause irritation. Cutting back on sugar can help you keep your skin fresh and healthy.

Processed meals: The harmful fats, carbohydrates, and additives included in processed meals can have a detrimental effect on the health of your skin.

Dairy: According to certain research, some people may be more susceptible to acne and other skin conditions when they consume dairy products. For some people, experimenting with cutting back on or giving up dairy products may be helpful.

Natural Solutions for Optimal Skin Health:

Green Tea: Packed with antioxidants, green tea helps lessen inflammation and shield the skin from harm.

Aloe Vera: Well renowned for its calming qualities, aloe vera helps moisturize skin and lessen irritation.

Coconut Oil: Packed with good fats, coconut oil has moisturizing properties. the skin and lessen swelling.

In summary,

1. Clear, healthy skin can be encouraged by eating a balanced diet full of fruits, vegetables, complete grains, and lean meats.

2. Foods high in antioxidants, like spinach, oranges, and berries, can help shield skin cells from aging and damage.

3. Vitamin C-rich foods, such as bell peppers and citrus fruits, can increase the formation of collagen and improve the suppleness of the skin.

4. Omega-3 fatty acids, which are present in walnuts, flaxseeds, and seafood, can help moisturize and lessen inflammation in the skin.

5. Foods high in zinc, like oysters, almonds, and seeds, can help control oil production and stop acne outbreaks.

6. Maintaining hydration and drinking lots of water will help keep skin hydrated and enhance general skin health.

7. Antioxidants found in green tea can help shield skin from UV rays and lessen irritation and redness.

8. You can avoid skin problems like acne and early aging by avoiding processed foods, sugary snacks, and excessive alcohol.

9. Including foods high in probiotics, such as kefir and yogurt, can help balance gut flora and treat skin issues like acne and eczema.

10. Foods high in vitamin E, such spinach, sunflower seeds, and almonds, can help shield skin from damage brought on by free radicals.

11. Sulfur-rich foods, such onions, garlic, and cruciferous vegetables, can aid in reducing inflammation and boosting the formation of collagen.

12. Steer clear of allergic foods like dairy and Gluten has the potential to alleviate skin irritation and ameliorate ailments such as psoriasis and eczema.

13. Eating foods strong in beta-carotene, such as cantaloupe, sweet potatoes, and carrots, will help preserve the texture and tone of your skin.

14. Eating foods high in selenium, such as whole grains, eggs, and Brazil nuts, can help shield skin cells from aging and damage.

15. To sum up, eating a diet high in nutrient-dense foods can help to promote healthy, clear skin.

Diet is a major factor in supporting healthy, clear skin.

You can support skin health and keep a beautiful complexion by including foods high in nutrients in your diet and adhering to dietary guidelines for healthy skin.

chapter 15
Gut Health and Nutrition: The Gut-Brain Connection and Its Impact on Overall Health

Because of its complex network of neurons and capacity for communication with the central nervous system, the gut is frequently referred to as the "second brain". Numerous elements of health, including as digestion, mood management, immunological function, and even cognitive function, depend heavily on this gut-brain axis. This chapter delves into the correlation between gut health and nutrition, the function of the gut-brain axis in general health, and useful dietary recommendations for promoting gut health.

Comprehending Gut Health:

Trillions of bacteria make up the gut microbiota, which is essential to gut health.

There is a balance and diversity among the helpful and dangerous bacteria in the gut microbiota of a healthy individual.

The Brain-Gut Relationship:

The gut-brain axis connects the gut with the brain. an intricate network of communication that operates in both directions and is made up of the endocrine, intestinal, and central nervous systems.

Through this communication system, the gut can affect brain function and vice versa, affecting mood, behavior, and cognitive abilities, among other aspects of health.

Nutrition's Effect on Gut Health

One of the biggest variables influencing intestinal health is diet. While some food choices can support a balanced gut flora, others can upset it.

Foods high in fiber: Because fiber encourages the growth of good bacteria in the gut, it is vital for gut health. Nuts, whole grains, legumes, fruits, and vegetables are good sources of fiber.

Fermented foods: Fermented foods such as yogurt, kefir, sauerkraut, kimchi, and kombucha include probiotics, helpful microorganisms that assist digestive wellness.

foods high in prebiotics: Prebiotics are indigestible fibers that nourish good bacteria in the digestive system. Bananas, asparagus, leeks, garlic, and onions are foods high in prebiotics.

Foods high in polyphenols: Berries, green tea, red wine, and dark chocolate are foods high in polyphenols, which are known to have antioxidant qualities and to promote intestinal health.

Gut Health's Effect on General Health Digestive health: Correct digestion and nutrient absorption depend on a healthy gut bacterium.

immunological function: In order to fight off infections and inflammation, the gut microbiota is essential to immunological function.

Mood regulation: Disorders related to anxiety, depression, and stress are associated to disturbances in gut health. This shows how the gut-brain relationship affects mood and emotional well-being.

Cognitive function: New study indicates that the gut microbiota may affect brain health and cognitive function, which may have consequences for diseases like Parkinson's and Alzheimer's.

Useful Advice for Promoting Gut Health

Consume a wide variety of foods high in fiber, such as nuts, legumes, whole grains, fruits, and vegetables.

Consume fermented foods on a daily basis to help your gut grow good bacteria.

Eat meals high in prebiotics to give you energy. for the gut's healthy microorganisms.

Eat less processed food, sweetened drinks, and artificial sweeteners as these can cause digestive problems.

Use stress-reduction methods including yoga, meditation, deep breathing exercises, and time spent in nature.

Specific Health Conditions and Gut Health:

Irritable bowel syndrome (IBS): low-FODMAP or high-fiber diets are frequently advised, as gut dysbiosis and inflammation are prominent symptoms of IBS.

Chronic inflammation of the digestive system is a hallmark of Crohn's disease, ulcerative colitis, and inflammatory bowel disease (IBD). Diet plays a part in managing symptoms and the course of the disease.

Obesity: Dietary therapies like fiber-rich diets and probiotic supplements show promise for managing weight. The gut microbiota composition may differ in obese persons.

Disorders related to mental health:

There may be a connection between gut health and mental health conditions like anxiety, depression, and autism spectrum disorders, according to emerging studies. In certain situations, dietary changes and probiotic supplements may be helpful.

In summary

Gut health is essential to general health and wellbeing since it affects immunological response, mood management, digestion, and cognitive performance.

People can optimize their gut flora and enhance general health and vitality by practicing mindful eating and promoting gut health through nutrition.

Chapter 16
Cooking and Food Preparation Skills: Fundamental Cooking Techniques for Nutritious Dinners

First of all,

Cooking is a fun and creative activity that can encourage healthier eating habits in addition to being a required skill for meal preparation. This chapter covers fundamental cooking skills for making healthful meals, such as necessary cooking methods, kitchenware, and advice on organizing and preparing meals.

Crucial Cooking Methods:

Knife Skills: To prepare materials quickly and securely, become proficient in fundamental knife skills like chopping, dicing, and mincing.
Sauteing is the process of swiftly frying food at high heat in a tiny amount of oil. It is a flexible cooking method that works well with meats, fish, and vegetables.
Roasting: Roasting is the process of cooking food at a high temperature in an oven. It is a dry-heat cooking technique that improves the texture and flavor of meats, poultry, and vegetables.
Boiling and Steaming: Boiling is the process of cooking food in a liquid, like broth or water; steaming is the process of cooking food over hot water. Seafood, cereals, and veggies work best with both techniques.
Cooking meals over an open flame or other heat source is known as grilling. It's an A cooking technique that can give vegetables, poultry, and meats a smokey flavor.
Kitchen Utensils and Provisions:

Knives: For effective meal preparation, choose a collection of premium knives that includes a chef's knife, paring knife, and serrated knife.
Cutting Boards: To safeguard your counters and avoid cross-contamination, choose cutting boards composed of plastic or wood.
Pots and Pans: Most culinary needs can be met with a simple collection of pots and pans that includes a stockpot, saute pan, and saucepan.
Cutlery: A spatula, tongs, whisk, and ladle are necessary kitchen tools for preparing and serving food.
Measuring Tools: To precisely measure ingredients for recipes, use measuring spoons and cups.

Tips for Meal Planning and Preparation:

Make a Plan: Set aside time to organize your weekly menu, which should include breakfast, lunch, dinner, and snacks. By doing this, you may cut down on food waste and save time and money.
Create a List for Your Shopping: To prevent impulsive purchases, make a shopping list based on your food plan and follow it.
Prepare Ahead: To save time during the week, prepare things ahead of time, such as chopping vegetables or marinating meats.
Cooking in batches: Make a lot of food in advance and portion it out into freezer-safe pieces for quick and simple meals all week long.
Utilize Leftovers: Turn leftovers into new dishes by adding leftover chicken to a salad or stir-fry, for example.

Tips for Healthy Cooking:

Use Healthful Cooking Techniques: To cut calories, choose cooking techniques like baking, roasting, steaming, and grilling that require less fat.
Select Whole Foods: For extra nourishment, include

entire foods in your meals, such as fruits, vegetables, whole grains, and lean proteins.
Minimize Salt and Sugar: Instead of adding salt and sugar to your food, flavor it using herbs, spices, and citrus juices.
Try Different Herbs & Spices: To enhance the flavor of your food without adding extra calories or sodium, use a range of herbs and spices.
Consider Portion Sizes: To stay within a healthy weight range and prevent overindulging, pay attention to portion sizes.
In summary:
Being able to cook is a useful skill that will enable you to make tasty and nutritious meals at home. You can reap the benefits of eating at home and enhance your general health and well-being by learning basic culinary techniques, using the appropriate tools and equipment, and planning and preparing meals in advance.

chapter 17:
Smart Snacking: Nutritious Snack Options for Long-Term Energy

First of all,

Smart snacking is a vital element of a healthy diet, giving energy and minerals between meals. This chapter examines the advantages of making wise snack choices, offers advice on selecting healthful snacks, and provides a range of wholesome snack suggestions to keep you feeling full all day.

Advantages of Strategic Snacking

Gives Energy: Between meals, snacks can assist sustain energy levels, particularly on hectic days or during physical activity.
Prevents Overeating: By reducing hunger and managing portion sizes, mindful snacking helps avoid overindulging during mealtimes.
Boosts Nutrient Intake: Fiber, vitamins, and minerals are just a few of the nutrients that a healthy snack can help you get in each day.
Promotes Weight Management: By limiting your calorie consumption, nutrient-dense snack choices can assist you in keeping a healthy weight.
Look for Whole Foods: Select snacks like fruits, vegetables, nuts, and seeds that are prepared from whole, minimally processed components.
Verify the Labels: Steer clear of snacks that are heavy in artificial chemicals, bad fats, and added sweets. Seek for snacks that have easily recognized, basic ingredients.
Think About Portion Sizes Take note of serving sizes to prevent overindulging. To manage portion proportions,

use tiny bowls or containers.
Macronutrient balance: To provide you lasting energy, pick snacks that are balanced in terms of carbs, protein, and healthy fats.
Maintain Hydration: Throughout the day, stay hydrated as much as possible because occasionally, thirst might be confused with hunger.
Ideas for Healthful Snacks:
Fruit and Nut Butter: For a filling and healthy snack, slice an apple or banana and spread peanut butter or almond butter on top.
Greek Yogurt Parfait: For a high-protein, high-fiber, and high-antioxidant snack, layer Greek yogurt with granola and mixed berries.
Hummus & Carrots: Dice up raw veggies like bell peppers, carrots, and cucumbers, then pair them with hummus to make a crisp and filling snack.
Trail Mix: For a tasty and sweet snack, mix nuts, seeds, dried fruit, and dark chocolate chips in your own trail mix.
Whole Grain Crackers and Cheese: For a filling and well-balanced snack, use whole grain crackers and a slice of cheese.
Popcorn: For a flavorful, low-calorie snack, air-pop popcorn and sprinkle it with sea salt and nutritional yeast.
Rice Cake with Avocado: For an easy and filling snack, top a rice cake with mashed avocado, a dash of salt and pepper, and a drizzle of olive oil.
Concise Snacking on the Run:
Look for Whole Foods: Choose snacks that are made from whole, minimally processed ingredients, such as fruits, vegetables, nuts, and seeds. Check the Labels: Avoid snacks that are high in added sugars, unhealthy fats, and artificial ingredients. Look for snacks with

simple, recognizable ingredients. Consider Portion Sizes: Pay attention to portion sizes to avoid overeating. Use small bowls or containers to control portion sizes. Balance Macronutrients: Choose snacks that contain a balance of carbohydrates, protein, and healthy fats to provide sustained energy. Stay Hydrated: Drink plenty of water throughout the day, as dehydration can sometimes be mistaken for hunger. Healthy Snack Ideas: Pack Portable Snacks: Prepare snacks ahead of time and pack them in small containers or zip-top bags for easy, on-the-go snacking.

Choose Convenience: Look for healthy, pre-packaged snacks, such as whole grain crackers, string cheese, or single-serve nut butter packets, for quick and easy snacking. Plan Ahead: Anticipate when you'll need a snack and plan accordingly to avoid unhealthy vending machine options or fast food. Conclusion: Smart snacking can help you maintain energy levels, prevent overeating, and boost nutrient intake. By choosing healthy, balanced snacks and planning ahead, you can enjoy the benefits of smart snacking and support your overall health and well-being.

Chapter 18
Hydration: The Importance of Water and Staying Hydrated

Introduction:
Hydration is essential for overall health and well-being, as water plays a crucial role in many bodily functions. This chapter explores the importance of hydration, the signs of dehydration, tips for staying hydrated, and the benefits of drinking enough water for optimal health.

The Importance of Hydration:
Water is essential for life and makes up a significant portion of the human body, including blood, cells, and tissues. Hydration is important for maintaining body temperature, lubricating joints, transporting nutrients and waste, and supporting digestion and metabolism.

Signs of Dehydration: Thirst: Feeling thirsty is the body's way of signaling that it needs more water. Dark Urine: Dark yellow or amber-colored urine is a sign of dehydration. In a well-hydrated person, urine is pale yellow. Fatigue: Dehydration can lead to fatigue and low energy levels. Dry Skin and Mouth: Dehydration can cause dry skin, lips, and mouth. Headache: Lack of water can lead to headaches and dizziness. Factors Affecting Hydration Needs:

Activity Level: Physical activity increases the body's need for water, as sweating and breathing can lead to fluid loss. Climate: Hot and humid weather can increase the risk of dehydration, as the body loses more water through sweating. Age: Infants, children, and older adults are at a higher risk of dehydration due to their smaller body size or decreased thirst sensation. Tips for Staying Hydrated: Drink Water Regularly: Aim to drink water throughout the day, rather than waiting until you feel thirsty. Carry a Water Bottle: Keep a reusable water bottle with you to remind yourself to drink water

regularly. Eat Water-Rich Foods: Include fruits and vegetables with high water content, such as watermelon, cucumber, and oranges, in your diet.
Limit Caffeine and Alcohol: Caffeine and alcohol can have a diuretic effect, increasing fluid loss. Limit your intake of these beverages and drink water instead. Monitor Urine Color: Check the color of your urine regularly. If it is dark yellow, drink more water. Benefits of Staying Hydrated: Improved Physical Performance: Staying hydrated can improve athletic performance and reduce fatigue during exercise. Better Digestion: Water is essential for digestion, helping to dissolve nutrients and transport them to cells. Clearer Skin: Adequate hydration can help maintain skin elasticity and promote a clear complexion. Weight Management: Drinking water before meals can help reduce calorie intake and support weight loss efforts. Hydration and Health Conditions:

Kidney Stones: Staying hydrated can reduce the risk of kidney stones by diluting the concentration of minerals in the urine. Urinary Tract Infections: Drinking plenty of water can help flush out bacteria from the urinary tract, reducing the risk of infection. Constipation: Adequate hydration is important for maintaining regular bowel movements and preventing constipation. Conclusion: Hydration is essential for overall health and well-being, supporting various bodily functions and promoting optimal health. By drinking water regularly, monitoring urine color, and incorporating water-rich foods into your diet, you can stay hydrated and enjoy the many benefits of proper hydration.

chapter 19
Eating Out Healthily: Making Healthy Choices

When Dining Out or Ordering In Introduction:

Eating out or ordering in can be a challenge when trying to maintain a healthy diet. However, with some planning and awareness, it is possible to make healthier choices that support your overall health and well-being. This chapter explores strategies for eating out healthily, including tips for navigating restaurant menus, making mindful choices, and managing portion sizes. Plan Ahead: Research Restaurants: Look up menus online before going out to choose restaurants that offer healthy options. Check Reviews: Read reviews to find restaurants that prioritize fresh, healthy ingredients and offer balanced meals. Have a Snack: Eating a small, healthy snack before going out can help prevent overeating when faced with a tempting menu.

Navigate the Menu:

Look for Keywords: Choose menu items that are grilled, baked, steamed, or roasted, as these cooking methods are generally healthier than fried or breaded options. Opt for Lean Proteins: Choose lean protein sources, such as grilled chicken, fish, or tofu, instead of fried or fatty meats. Load Up on Vegetables: Order dishes that are rich in vegetables or ask for extra vegetables as a side. Watch Out for Hidden Calories: Be cautious of dishes that are high in hidden calories, such as creamy sauces, dressings, or cheese. Make Mindful Choices: Listen to Your Body: Pay attention to your hunger and fullness cues and stop eating when you are satisfied, rather than finishing everything on your plate. Practice Portion Control: Consider sharing a meal with a How to Use the Menu:

Treat Yourself Sometimes: It's acceptable to treat

yourself to your favorite foods once in a while, but make an effort to balance it out with healthier options during the week.

Savor the Moment: Savor your meal and socialize with others without feeling guilty because dining out should be enjoyable.

In summary:

With some preparation, awareness, and wise decisions, eating out may be done in a healthful manner. You can enjoy delectable meals and interacting with friends and family while making healthy choices while dining out or ordering in by using these guidelines.

chapter 20
Understanding the Physical and Mental Benefits of Exercise and Its Role in Health

First of all,

Exercise provides numerous advantages for both physical and mental health, making it an essential part of a healthy lifestyle. This chapter examines the benefits of exercise for general health, including how it affects quality of life, disease prevention, physical fitness, and mental health.

Benefits of Exercise on the Body:

Better Cardiovascular Health: Engaging in regular exercise helps lower blood pressure, strengthen the heart muscle, and improve circulation, all of which lessen the risk of heart disease and stroke.
Weight Management: Exercise is a key component in managing weight and preventing obesity because it burns calories and helps build muscle.
Enhanced Endurance and Muscle Strength: Strength training activities can assist increase total strength and muscle mass.
and stamina.
Increased Flexibility and Balance: Especially for older persons, stretching exercises can help increase flexibility and balance, which lowers the risk of falls and accidents.
Prevention of Diseases:
Lower Risk of Chronic Diseases: Engaging in regular exercise helps lower the risk of developing or managing long-term health issues like osteoporosis, diabetes, and hypertension.

Enhanced Immune Response: Physical activity can strengthen the immune system, lowering the chance of infections and diseases.

Cancer Prevention: Research indicates that engaging in regular physical activity may lower the chance of developing certain cancers, such as colon and breast cancer.

Advantages for Mental Health:

Decreased Anxiety and Stress: Exercise is a natural way to relieve stress since it causes the release of endorphins, which lift your spirits and lessen anxiety and tension.

Better Sleep: Getting regular exercise can help you get better sleep and lower your risk of developing sleep problems like insomnia.

Exercise has been associated with enhanced cognitive function, including enhanced memory, attention, and general cognitive performance, which lowers the risk of aging-related cognitive deterioration.

Improved Mental Health: Physical activity can help reduce depressive symptoms and enhance mental health in general.

Life Quality:

Selecting rituals that you can realistically integrate into your everyday life and that you find meaningful is vital when building daily routines. The following advice can help you establish meaningful daily routines:

Start modest: Start by adding one or two easy daily rituals to your schedule. You can progressively add additional rituals as you get more accustomed to them.

To create a sense of habit and consistency, try practicing your rituals at the same time every day.

Make it your own: Your own hobbies, values, and preferences should all be reflected in your everyday routines. Select activities that are genuine and relevant to you.

Be adaptable: Being flexible and versatile is just as vital as maintaining consistency. Because life is erratic, there will be moments when It could be necessary for you to modify your rituals to account for evolving situations.

Try new things and make adjustments: Don't be scared to try out several routines to find which one suits you the best. You are welcome to modify or substitute a ritual if it is no longer serving you.

The Advantages of Daily Customs

Your physical, mental, and emotional health can all benefit greatly from establishing daily rituals. Among the advantages are:

Decreased stress and anxiety: Establishing daily routines can aid in your relaxation and make you feel less stressed and anxious.
Enhanced productivity and focus: Establishing daily rituals will help you start the day with clarity and focus, which will increase your output in general.
Improved well-being: Establishing daily routines might help you feel happier and more contented by elevating your mood and general sense of well-being.
Enhanced mindfulness: Establishing daily routines will help you develop an awareness and presence that will increase your enjoyment of the present.
In summary

Establishing regular routines might help people feel grounded and stable in a world that is always changing. Daily rituals, such as an evening stroll, an early morning meditation practice, or a gratitude notebook, can support you in setting goals for the day, staying focused and in balance during the day, and unwinding at the end of the day. Thus, invest some time in developing meaningful daily routines that suit your needs and reap the numerous advantages of establishing daily rituals in your life.

Chapter 21
Conscientious Time Management: Allocating Time for What Really Counts

Overview

Time is valuable in the fast-paced world of today. The demands of work, family, and personal obligations can make it seem as though there is never enough time in the day to complete everything. You may, however, learn to prioritize your most important tasks and make the most use of your time by engaging in mindful time management practices. We will examine the idea of conscious time management in this chapter, along with its significance and practical applications.

Comprehending Conscientious Time Management

Effective time management involves more than just finishing tasks; it also entails using your time with intention and awareness. It entails monitoring how you spend your time, making Establish Your Objectives: Decide if your goal for your workout program is to reduce weight, grow muscle, increase fitness, or relieve stress.

Have Reasonable Expectations: To keep yourself motivated, set attainable objectives that are time-bound, precise, and measurable.

Think About Your Preferences:

Think About Your Interests: List the pursuits you find enjoyable or have always wanted to pursue, such as yoga, hiking, swimming, or dance.

Mix It Up: Adding variety to your workout regimen will help you stay engaged and avoid boredom. Explore a variety of pursuits to determine your favorite.
Determine Your Degree of Fitness:
Start Slow: As your fitness level increases, progressively increase the intensity of your low-impact exercise regimen. This is especially important if you're new to exercising or returning to it after a break.
Pay Attention to Your Body: Observe your body's reaction to exercise and recovery. If something doesn't feel right, halt and consult a medical expert for help.
Try Various Tasks:

Examine Your Choices: Explore a range of pursuits to discover your passions. To determine what works best for you, try group programs, outdoor activities, or at-home workouts.
Maintain an Open Mind: Never be scared to attempt new things. You can develop a strong interest in a previously unconsidered hobby.
Make It Social
Workout with Friends: Joining a group fitness class or working out with friends might help you stay motivated and enjoy your workouts more.
Join a Community: Participating in sports or fitness classes can foster a sense of support and community that enhances the enjoyment of exercise.
Establish a Timetable:

Make Working Out a Priority: To make sure you make time for exercise, schedule your exercises just as you would any other appointment.
Be Adaptable: Since life is unpredictable, be prepared to change your plans when needed. Keep in mind that any

activity is better than none at all.

Make It Enjoyable:

Play music: To stay inspired and motivated while working out, compile a playlist of your best tunes. Give yourself a reward when you reach your modest objectives. This can support your motivation and involvement in your workout regimen.

Remain Steady:

Create a Routine: Choose an exercise regimen that works for your lifestyle and schedule. Making exercise a habit and observing results require consistency. Monitor Your Development: To stay motivated and observe your progress, keep a record of your workouts and accomplishments.

In summary:

The secret to maintaining a fitness regimen over time is to find one you enjoy. You may identify pleasant, sustainable activities that support your fitness goals by taking your preferences, goals, and degree of fitness into account.

Never forget that working out should be enjoyable and fulfilling, so don't be scared to try new things and modify your regimen as necessary.

chapter 22
Overcoming Exercise Barriers: Dealing with Typical Challenges to Maintaining an Active Lifestyle

First of all,

Frequent exercise is crucial for preserving health and wellbeing, yet staying active can be difficult for many people due to various challenges. In order to help you create and stick to an exercise regimen that suits you, this chapter examines various obstacles to exercise and offers solutions.

Insufficient Time:
Exercise should be prioritized, therefore plan it into your schedule just like any other appointment.
Cut Down on Workouts: If you're pressed for time, concentrate on quick, intense workouts that take no more than 30 minutes to do.
Include Exercise in Your Daily Routine: Seek for opportunities to move during the day, like going for a stroll during your lunch break or choosing to use the stairs rather than the elevator.
Absence of drive:

Make definite, attainable goals to help you stay motivated to get out on a regular basis.
Locate a Partner for Accountability: Joining a group exercise class or working out with a friend might help you stay accountable and motivated.
Mix It Up: To keep things fresh and avoid monotony, try a variety of exercises.
Experiencing Fear or Feeling Overburdened:

Start Slow: As your confidence and fitness grow, start with low-intensity exercises and progressively up the ante.

Seek Support: To help you feel more at ease with exercise, think about working with a personal trainer or fitness coach.

Remind yourself that everyone begins somewhere, and that the most crucial thing to do is to keep your attention on your own development and objectives.

Physical Restraints:

Speak with a Healthcare expert: Before beginning a new workout regimen, get advice from a healthcare expert if you have any physical restrictions or health issues.

Select Low-Impact Exercises: Think about low-impact exercises that are easier on the joints, like yoga, cycling, or swimming.

Adjust the Exercises: Exercises should be adjusted to your comfort level and skill level. For instance, you can carry out strength training activities while seated if It is difficult to stand.

Inability to Access Equipment or Facilities:

Wear Proper Clothes: To make exercising outside more comfortable, spend money on clothes that are appropriate for the various weather situations.

Maintain a Plan B: In the event of bad weather, keep an alternate indoor fitness regimen handy, such as an indoor cycling program or an exercise DVD.

Acknowledge the Seasons: To add some spice to your workout regimen, try trying some seasonal sports like swimming in the summer or skiing in the winter.

Budgetary Restrictions:

Look for Low-Cost Options: A lot of places have free or inexpensive sports leagues, walking clubs, and fitness programs.

DIY Fitness: For at-home workouts that require little to no equipment, use online resources like fitness apps or workout videos.

Negotiate Prices: To make a gym membership or fitness class more affordable, ask about discounts or payment options. Getting beyond obstacles to exercise is crucial to starting and keeping up a regular exercise schedule.

You may incorporate regular exercise into your life and reap the numerous health and well-being benefits it provides by addressing common hurdles and putting measures in place to overcome them.

chapter 23
Establishing a Lifestyle that Encourages Good Food and Exercise Habits and Creating a Supportive Environment

First of all,

Maintaining healthy food and exercise habits depends on having a supportive environment. This chapter discusses how to create a lifestyle that supports healthy choices, including how to arrange your home, office, and social circle to support your fitness and health objectives.

Establish Specific Objectives:

No. Topic Information 1. Stocking Your Kitchen with Healthful Foods: Make sure your kitchen is stocked with whole grains, fruits, veggies, and lean proteins. 2. Cooking Healthful Meal. To ensure you have wholesome meals and snacks on hand when you need them, prepare them ahead of time.
3. Establishing an Exercise Area Set aside a room in your house for exercising, such as a tiny home gym or a yoga nook.
4. Including Your Emotions Invite your family to follow your example of a balanced diet and regular exercise.
5. Bringing Nutritious Food to Work To avoid the unhealthy cafeteria alternatives, bring your own nutritious meals and snacks to work.
6. Taking Regular Breaks at Work Arrange for short workouts, walks, or stretches during the day.
7. Promoting Well-Being at Work Encourage your employer to implement workplace wellness initiatives, such as standing desks or exercise challenges.

8. Assembling a Supportive Group of People Create a support system of sociable people in your wholesome lifestyle decisions.
9. Arranging Engaging Activities Arrange physical activities-focused events like riding, dancing, or hiking.
10. Sharing Your Objectives To get support and accountability, tell your friends and family about your exercise and health objectives.
11. Making Self-Compassion a Practice, If you falter or have setbacks in your healthy behaviors, treat yourself with kindness.
12. Having Reasonable Expectations Establish long-term, attainable goals that you can stick with.
13. Putting Progress Above Perfection Recognize your advancement and celebrate your accomplishments, no matter how tiny.
14. Creating a Daily Schedule Establish a schedule that allows for self-care, exercise, and wholesome meals.
15. Developing Healthful Habits Small at First One good habit at a time, start small, and add more as you go.
16. Setting Aside Time to Work Out Include frequent workouts in your weekly schedule.
17. Building an At-Home Workout Make a specific area in your house for your workout gear.
18. Promoting Physical Exercise at Work Promote strolling gatherings or active intermissions during the working day.
19. Including Exercise in Everyday Tasks Seek out opportunities to move during the day, like walking or using the stairs to run errands.
20. Attending Group Exercise Courses For motivation and social support, sign up for group exercise programs or sports teams.

Establish Your Objectives: Set attainable, measurable goals for yourself that are consistent with your beliefs and values regarding exercise and a healthy diet.
Break It Down: To make larger goals more attainable and to monitor your progress along the way, break them down into smaller, more manageable steps.
Establish a Healthful Atmosphere at Home:

Stock Up on Nutritious Foods: To facilitate healthy eating, stock your kitchen with foods high in vitamins, minerals, whole grains, and lean proteins.
Prepare Ahead: To ensure that you have wholesome meals and snacks on hand for when hunger strikes, prepare them in advance.
Minimize Temptations: To lessen the temptation to overindulge in unhealthy meals, keep them hidden from view or out of the house.
Make Working Out Convenient:

Pick a Convenient Location: To make it simpler to fit exercise into your schedule, choose a gym or fitness center that is close to your house or place of employment.
Maintain a Backup Plan: If you can't work out on a given day, have a fallback plan in place, such watching an exercise DVD or taking a stroll around the neighborhood.
Plan Frequent Exercises: Make exercise a non-negotiable part of your day and schedule it into your calendar like you would any important appointment.
Embrace a Supportive Social Circle:

Find People Who Share Your Thoughts: Join a club, class, or fitness group to meet people who have similar fitness and health objectives.

Ask Friends and Family for Assistance: Ask your loved ones and friends to help you achieve your goals for their assistance in assisting you in reaching them.

Steer Clear of Negative Influences: Keep your distance from people who could undermine your efforts or promote bad habits.

Create a Helpful Work Environment: Incorporate brief, dynamic breaks into your workday by doing things like going for a walk during lunch or setting up a standing desk.

Promote Healthier Decisions: Promote workplace regulations that encourage physical activity and a healthy diet, such as those that offer gym memberships or healthy snack options.

Establish a Culture of Support: Encourage the development of a healthy work environment where employees feel supported and encouraged to make healthy decisions.

Control Stress and Make Self-Care a Priority:

Use Stress-Reduction Strategies: Include stress-reduction practices in your everyday routine, such as yoga, meditation, or deep breathing exercises.

Set priorities. Rest: To promote your general health and well-being, make sure you receive enough good sleep every night.

Set Aside Time for Yourself: Plan regular self-care activities to help you unwind, read, or engage in hobbies lessen tension.

Honor accomplishments and draw lessons from failures:

Incorporate brief, dynamic breaks into your workday by doing things like going for a walk during lunch or setting up a standing desk.

Promote Healthier Decisions: Promote workplace

regulations that encourage physical activity and a healthy diet, such as those that offer gym memberships or healthy snack options.
Establish a Culture of Support: Encourage the development of a healthy work environment where employees feel supported and encouraged to make healthy decisions.
Control Stress and Make Self-Care a Priority:

Use Stress-Reduction Strategies: Include stress-reduction practices in your everyday routine, such as yoga, meditation, or deep breathing exercises.
Set priorities. Rest: To promote your general health and well-being, make sure you receive enough good sleep every night.
Set Aside Time for Yourself: Plan regular self-care activities to help you unwind, read, or engage in hobbies.

www.ingramcontent.com/pod-product-compliance
Lightning Source LLC
Chambersburg PA
CBHW070119230526
45472CB00004B/1332